101 TIPS FOR IMPROVING YOUR BLOOD SUGAR

▲

A project of the
American Diabetes Association

▼

Written by
The University of New Mexico
Diabetes Care Group

David S. Schade, MD, *Editor in Chief*

Patrick J. Boyle, MD

Mark R. Burge, MD

Carolyn Johannes, RN, CDE

Virginia Valentine, RN, MS, CDE

▲. American Diabetes Association.

Publisher
Susan H. Lau

Graphic Designer
Paul Akmajian, MFA

Editorial Director
Peter Banks

Editor
Sherrye Landrum

The "tips" in this book were developed from the authors' experience with the DCCT and are not official Position Statements or Clinical Practice Recommendations of the American Diabetes Association.

Printed in the United States of America

AMERICAN DIABETES ASSOCIATION
1660 Duke Street
Alexandria, Virginia 22314

Library of Congress Cataloging-in-Publication Data
101 Tips for improving your blood sugar: a project of the American Diabetes Association/written and produced by the University of New Mexico Diabetes Care Group; David S. Schade, M.D., editor in chief...[et al.].
p. cm.
Includes index.
ISBN 0-945448-47-3
I. Schade, David S., 1942-   . II. University of New Mexico.
Diabetes Care Group. III. American Diabetes Association.
RC660.4.A15   1995   95-9922
616.4'62--dc20   CIP

101 TIPS FOR IMPROVING YOUR BLOOD SUGAR

▼

TABLE OF CONTENTS

ACKNOWLEDGMENTS

▼

The University of New Mexico Diabetes Care Group wishes to acknowledge the talent, graphic design, and desktop publishing skills of Paul Akmajian, MFA, of the University of New Mexico. His skills brought this book to life. We also acknowledge the editorial assistance of Sherrye Landrum of the American Diabetes Association; the assistance of Carolyn King of the University of New Mexico; the artistic talent of Rebecca Grace Jones, and the graphic expertise of Steve Rhodes of Insight Graphics for the cover design. Thanks to Karen Ingle for copyediting and to David Kelley, MD, and Linda Lacey, RN, CDE, for reviewing the manuscript. Steve Shartel coordinated printing.

CONTRIBUTORS

▼

The University of New Mexico Diabetes Care Group:

David S. Schade, MD	Diabetes Specialist
Patrick J. Boyle, MD	Diabetes Specialist
Mark R. Burge, MD	Diabetes Specialist
Carolyn Johannes, RN, CDE	Certified Diabetes Educator
Virginia Valentine, RN, MS, CDE	Clinical Nurse Specialist/Diabetes
and Paul Akmajian, MFA	Graphic Designer

INTRODUCTION

▼

The treatment of diabetes has dramatically changed in the last 5 years. No longer is it acceptable to permit blood sugar to remain above normal in the person with diabetes. The medical consequences of high blood sugar are largely preventable when the blood sugar is kept in the normal range.

During the last 10 years we have been fortunate to care for many people with diabetes who made the commitment to improve their blood-sugar levels. Most of these individuals have achieved their goals, and in addition, told us how they did it. This book is a collection of their suggestions and experiences that we would like to pass on to you. We hope that many of these tips will apply to your lifestyle and help you control your blood sugar more easily.

— The University of New Mexico Diabetes Care Group

Chapter One:
GENERAL TIPS

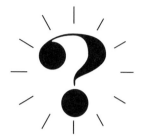 *H*ow *do I know if I have type I or type II diabetes?*

▼ TIP:

W ith type I diabetes the body stops making insulin. This usually occurs at a young age. People with type I diabetes will require insulin for life, because insulin is essential for using and storing food. These people are usually lean, and if they did not have insulin, would go into diabetic coma within a day or two. We call this disease, "Insulin-Dependent Diabetes Mellitus (IDDM)."

People with type II diabetes have enough insulin early in the disease but are unable to use the insulin correctly to lower their blood sugar. They are insulin resistant. Many people with type II diabetes are able to control their blood sugar with diet and exercise with or without oral diabetes pills. This type of diabetes is often called "Non-Insulin–Dependent Diabetes Mellitus (NIDDM)." After several years with type II diabetes, many of these people will need insulin, but they still have type II diabetes, insulin-requiring. Most people with type II diabetes are overweight and over 30 years old.

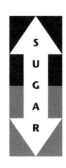

*W*hat was my average blood sugar before I got diabetes?

▼
TIP:

The answer to this question depends upon whether you have eaten food in the last 6 hours. Before breakfast, when you have not had food for 8 or more hours, your blood sugar would have been between 70 and 115 mg/dl. However, after you ate a meal, your sugar rose, but rarely went above 200 mg/dl. People who do not have diabetes don't have problems associated with high blood sugar (i.e., diabetic complications). That is why your blood-sugar goal is to stay close to the upper limit of normal blood-sugar ranges.

	Normal
Fasting blood sugar	<115mg/dl
(2-h) blood sugar	After meal 140mg/dl
Bedtime Glucose	<120mg/dl
Hemoglobin A_{1C}	<6%

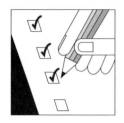

*W*hat are my blood-sugar goals if I have insulin-dependent *(type I)* diabetes?

TIP:

*W*e have slightly altered the American Diabetes Association recommendations for blood-sugar goals for people with type I diabetes. If you are having too many episodes of severe hypoglycemia (low blood sugar), raise your goal to the higher numbers. These goals are good general guidelines to help you measure your blood-sugar control.

Goals for People with Type I Diabetes

Before meal blood sugar	70–120 mg/dl
After meal blood sugar	< 180 mg/dl
Weekly average blood sugar	100–120 mg/dl
Urine ketones	absent
Hemoglobin A_{1C}	5.5–7%

(See Tips on page 28 and page 100.)

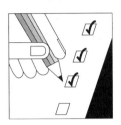

*W*hat are my blood sugar goals if I have non-insulin–dependent (**type II**) diabetes?

TIP:

*W*e encourage you to try for nearly normal blood-sugar levels with few episodes of low blood sugar. The American Diabetes Association (ADA) goals are listed below. If you are having too many low blood sugars, try the Acceptable range for a time, and then go for the ADA goals.

Goals for People with Type II Diabetes

	ADA Goals	Acceptable	Poor
Fasting blood sugar	70–120	140	>200 mg/dl
After meal (2-h) blood sugar	<180	200	>235 mg/dl
Glycosylated hemoglobin	<7%	8%	>10%
Hemoglobin A$_{1C}$	5.5–7%	7%	>9%

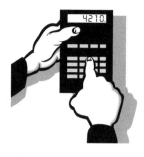

*H*ow can I tell if my diabetes program is successful?

▼
TIP:

K eep track of your diabetes the same way you do your checking account—by keeping tabs on the balance. With diabetes, the balance is the sum of

- Your blood sugar,
- Your weight,
- Your blood pressure,
- Your exercise, and
- How you feel.

If all of these items meet your goals, then you are doing fine.

Keep a daily record of your blood glucose, feelings, and exercise, and weekly or monthly records of your weight and blood pressure. Check your blood pressure at home or have it done at shopping centers, pharmacies, etc. Make daily exercise one of your goals. When you monitor your health, you help yourself succeed.

EXAMPLE RECORD

Date	Wt	Blood Pressure	Avg Glucose	Feelings	Exercise
6/1	150	122/80	102	Good	Yes
6/2	151	120/75	111	Good	No
6/3	149	115/80	98	So/So	Yes
etc.	etc.	etc.	etc.	etc.	etc.

*H*ow *can I save money while taking care of my diabetes?*

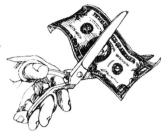

▼
TIP:

T aking good care of your diabetes is expensive. A large part of the expense goes for the supplies that you need to inject insulin and to monitor your blood sugar. Recently, generic test strips have become available for some glucose meters. You'll find a list of these strips in the October issue of *Forecast* magazine (or the annual ADA *Buyer's Guide*).

In addition, many patients use a new syringe and a new alcohol pad to clean their skin each time they inject insulin. This is not necessary. You can reuse your syringe, although the needle tip will begin to get dull after five injections. (Be sure to keep the needle tip clean and capped.) Alcohol pads are not necessary as long as the skin is cleaned with soap and water.

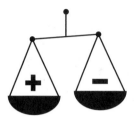

If I follow all the advice in this book and my blood-sugar control improves, are there drawbacks that I should be aware of?

▼
TIP:

Yes, there are. However, these are usually not bad enough to discourage you from keeping your blood sugar near normal. The two main concerns are frequent low blood sugar reactions and a tendency to gain weight. You can head off low blood sugar by monitoring carefully. You can keep your weight in line by watching the number of calories you eat and by increasing the amount of exercise you do. Overall, the disadvantages are minor compared to the benefits you gain from lowering your blood sugar.

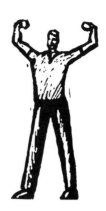

*W*hy should I work so hard to improve my
blood-sugar level?

▼
TIP:

B ecause you'll feel more energy and a sense of well-being
when your blood sugar enters the normal range. In addition, you'll delay or prevent problems with your eyes, kidneys, and nerves as your blood sugar improves. Many doctors also believe that problems with heart disease, strokes, and hardening of the arteries may be delayed by good blood-sugar control. If you do not get any complications of diabetes, you'll live a longer, healthier life.

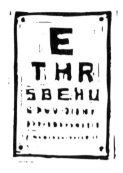

Will controlling my blood sugar prevent my recently diagnosed diabetic eye disease from getting worse?

TIP:

Yes. Although improving your blood-sugar control may temporarily make your eye disease worse, over the long term, it will help. The Diabetes Control and Complications Trial (DCCT) monitored patients with mild diabetic eye disease for years. This study showed that the diabetic eye disease of patients with good blood-sugar control progressed much more slowly than the eye disease of similar patients with poor blood-sugar control. This is a major reason to strive for excellent blood-sugar control, particularly if you have mild to moderate complications of diabetes.

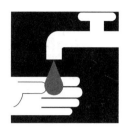

*D*o I have to use alcohol on my finger before checking my blood sugar like the nurses at the hospital do?

▼
TIP:

No. Using alcohol is not necessary before checking your blood-sugar level. Washing and drying your hands is enough. Test strips for checking the glucose (blood sugar) in your blood have a substance in them that causes sugar to turn into a colored chemical. Alcohol can destroy this substance and give you a false low blood-sugar reading. Alcohol is drying and can lead to broken skin near nails. Also, if all the alcohol doesn't evaporate before you stick your finger, you may feel stinging as well as the discomfort of the poke.

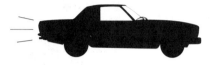

How should I prepare for a long car trip alone so I don't get high or low blood sugars?

▼
TIP:

The best way to approach a long driving trip alone is to establish a routine. Start your day early so that you can arrive at your destination early. Because you are less active while driving, exercise before you leave or stop along the way at a park or rest area and take a walk. You might also consider either slightly increasing your daily insulin or decreasing the amount of food that you eat. Because hypoglycemia (low blood sugar) is particularly dangerous when you are driving, plan on checking your blood-sugar levels frequently (every 2 to 4 hours) and always have some form of sugar in the car with you. Choose something that won't melt and mess up the upholstery in your car, such as glucose tablets, a bottle of regular soda, or vanilla wafers.

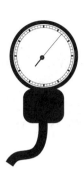

Why did my doctor recently start me on a blood pressure medication even though my blood pressure is only slightly elevated?

▼
TIP:

High blood sugar combined with high blood pressure increases your risk of getting diabetic kidney disease. Kidney disease can lead to kidney failure and the need for either dialysis or a kidney transplant. Doctors can identify diabetic kidney disease at a very early stage, when small amounts of protein appear in the urine (microalbuminuria). Certain drugs, such as ACE inhibitors, that lower blood pressure also lower microalbuminuria and can slow down the development of diabetic kidney disease.

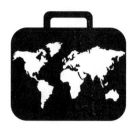

What if my blood glucose meter quits working while I am on an out-of-town trip?

▼
TIP:

Continue monitoring your blood sugar with visual test strips (Chemstrip, Diascan, Glucostix). These are available without a prescription at most pharmacies. In the meantime, call the toll-free number that can usually be found on the back of the meter. Most companies will try to replace the meter within a day or two.

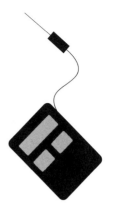

*W*ill an insulin pump improve my blood-sugar control?

▼
TIP:

M aybe, maybe not. It depends on the individual. These devices require you to pay close attention to your blood-sugar levels and to adjust your insulin, food, and exercise to achieve good readings. With an insulin pump, you can vary your mealtime schedule more readily than with insulin injections and you can skip a meal when you must. There is more flexibility for people with unpredictable mealtimes. Discuss the pros and cons of using an insulin pump and whether you are a good candidate for having one with your health-care team before purchasing one. Also, because they are expensive, check whether your insurance company will help cover the cost.

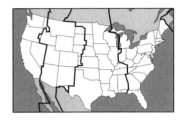

How do I make adjustments in my insulin when I travel across several time zones?

▼
TIP:

The easiest approach is to omit your intermediate- or long-acting insulin on the morning of the trip and rely on regular insulin to keep your blood sugar normal. You will have to test your blood sugar frequently (every 4 hours) and take regular insulin frequently (every 4 hours, adjusting the insulin dose to your blood-sugar level). When you arrive at your destination and change your watch to the new time zone, go back to your usual insulin and meal schedule.

Is there a level of average blood sugar below which I do not have to worry about complications from diabetes?

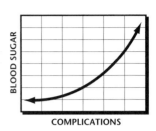

COMPLICATIONS

▼
TIP:

No. There is no "safe threshold." The Diabetes Control and Complications Trial (DCCT) looked at the relationship between average blood-sugar levels (measured by hemoglobin A_{1C}) and the beginning of complications. There is no level below which the risk disappears. However, the lower your hemoglobin A_{1C}, the lower your risk of eye, kidney, and nerve disease. Therefore, you should try for the best average blood sugar that you can (but avoid seriously low blood sugars) to reduce your risk of having diabetic complications.

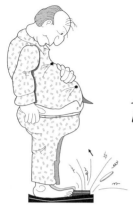

*H*ow does the fact that I am overweight
affect my ability to obtain normal
blood sugars?

▼
TIP:

B eing overweight causes resistance to insulin. This means
that any insulin your body may make (or that you inject)
will have a hard time lowering your blood sugar. This makes it
difficult for you to control your blood sugar. In addition, being
overweight may raise your blood pressure, which makes you
prone to kidney disease and stroke. Being overweight may also
be associated with high blood fat levels, which make you sus-
ceptible to hardening of the arteries. If you reduce your weight,
your blood sugar and your health will improve.

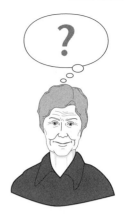

A t age 72, why should I worry about
blood-sugar control?

▼
TIP:

A ge alone is not a reason to ignore your diabetes control.
You may live to be 80 or 90. This is enough time for complications of diabetes to develop. The better your blood-sugar
control, the lower your risk of developing complications.

Some people are lowering their risk of diabetes complications through tight diabetes management. They do have
more frequent low blood sugar reactions, and that is riskier for
some people than for others. People with heart disease and
people who do not feel warning signs when they develop low
blood sugar (e.g., shakiness, sweating, increased heart rate)
need to be careful. Tight blood-sugar control is not for everyone (and may even be dangerous for some). You and your
health-care team should determine what blood-sugar levels are
right for you.

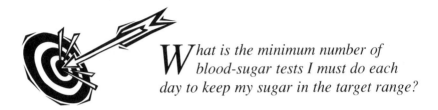

What is the minimum number of blood-sugar tests I must do each day to keep my sugar in the target range?

▼
TIP:

The answer depends on the type of diabetes you have. Most people with type I diabetes need to test their blood sugar four times a day (before each meal and at bedtime) to allow them to adjust their premeal insulin dose. People with type II diabetes may need to test only before breakfast each day. Occasionally, people with type I or type II diabetes should test their blood sugar 2–3 hours after a meal to find out if it is going too high or in the middle of the night to see if it is going too low. If it is, the amount of food, exercise, or medication may need to be adjusted. All people with diabetes should test their blood sugar any time they think it may be too high or too low. The symptoms of being high or low may be similar, or may not be due to blood sugar at all!

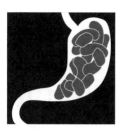

*W*ill *my blood-sugar level be affected if my stomach empties slowly?*

▼
TIP:

Yes. If it takes many hours for your stomach to empty and food to be absorbed, you risk low blood sugar when you take your insulin 45 minutes before you eat and high blood sugar hours after you eat when your stomach finally empties. The common cause of slowed digestion in people who have had diabetes for many years is damage to the nerves affecting stomach muscle motion. Unpredictable stomach emptying makes it difficult to achieve near normal blood sugars. There are several medications now available that may improve the motion of your stomach, and you should discuss these with your health-care team.

Chapter Two:
HIGH BLOOD SUGAR TIPS

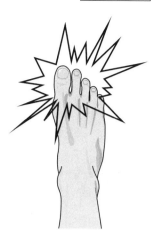

D *oes the pain in my feet have anything to do with high blood sugar?*

▼
TIP:

Probably. Especially if you have had high blood sugar and the pain has lasted for some time. Nerves work better when they are surrounded by normal rather than high blood sugar. Discuss your pain with your health-care team. Some people find the pain in their feet and legs will decrease when their blood sugar is brought closer to normal. Others find it painful for bedsheets to touch their feet. If you experience this, placing a hoop over the end of the bed so that the sheet is kept off of your feet will provide relief until your blood sugars can be lowered. If the problem doesn't go away with improved blood-sugar control, then putting capsaicin cream (which is made from chili peppers) on the affected skin may help. Other therapies are also available, so you need to discuss the various choices with your diabetes health-care team.

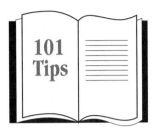

S ince I have read this book, why do I need help from anyone else to control my high blood sugars?

▼
TIP:

Although books on diabetes have many good, helpful suggestions to control your blood sugar, there are many situations in which additional advice is needed. Your doctor and health-care team can

1. Help you choose the blood-sugar goal that is appropriate for you,

2. Teach you how to care for your diabetes and keep you up-to-date on new treatments,

3. Help you develop a meal plan,

4. Check your medications so they don't interfere with each other,

5. Design a physical activity program specifically for you,

6. Review your blood-sugar records with you and make suggestions on how to improve your blood-sugar control, and

7. Help you manage your diabetes when you become ill and thereby prevent more serious health problems.

*W*hat *are the symptoms of high blood sugar?*

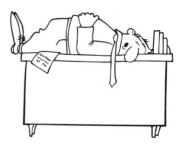

▼
TIP:

S ymptoms of high blood sugar may vary from person to person or even in one person from day to day. But, in general, a person will

1 Feel more hungry or thirsty than usual,

2 Have to urinate more frequently than normal,

3 Have to get up at night several times to go to the bathroom,

4 Feel very tired, sleepy, or have no energy, and

5 Be unable to see clearly or see "halos" when looking at a light.

If you have any of the above symptoms, locate your blood glucose meter and test immediately. Do not treat these symptoms with additional insulin unless you are certain that they are due to high blood sugar. Other conditions can cause similar symptoms.

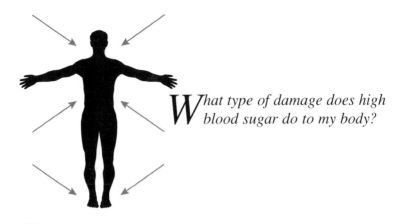

What type of damage does high blood sugar do to my body?

TIP:

High blood sugars over time can damage both blood vessels and nerves in your body. This can result in poor blood flow to your hands and feet in addition to your legs, arms, and vital organs. Poor blood flow to these areas increases your risk of infections, heart problems, stroke, blindness, foot or leg amputation, and kidney disease. In addition, you can either lose the feeling in your feet or have increased pain in your feet and legs. Damage to your feet can occur from mild trauma, and you may not know it. Finally, damage to blood vessels and nerves can lead to sexual problems that are difficult to treat. For all these reasons, you should make a major effort to avoid high blood sugars in your body.

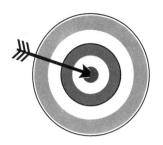

*W*hy is my glycosylated hemoglobin high when my average blood sugar is in my target range?

▼
TIP:

Your average blood sugar is based on your premeal blood sugars. While this usually works well, it does not take into account the level of your blood sugar after you eat. It may be that your blood sugar is rising unexpectedly after your meal because you are either not taking enough insulin or not taking insulin far enough ahead of eating your meal. To see if this is the reason that your glycosylated hemoglobin is high, measure your blood sugar level 2 hours after breakfast, lunch, and dinner for several days (in addition to your premeal blood sugars). Blood sugar over 200 mg/dl 2 hours after meals is too high. In addition, your blood sugar may be high throughout the night, when you are asleep. To find out, wake yourself up between 2 and 4:00 a.m. several times during the week to check your blood sugar. At 4:00 a.m., blood sugar over 150 mg/dl is too high. Continue to check your blood sugar 2 hours after meals and in the middle of the night once a month to be certain that you are not having unexpected high blood sugars at these times.

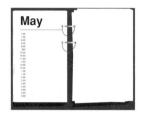

How can I evaluate my blood sugar control when my doctor does a hemoglobin A_{1C} only every 6 months?

▼
TIP:

You can use your self blood glucose test results to predict your hemoglobin A_{1C} (HbA_{1C}). Here's how. Average all your blood-sugar test results each week. (Our patients tested four times a day, but even one test a day will help you make a guess.) Find your average on the table below. Read across to the HbA_{1C} number. This will give you an idea of your HbA_{1C} range, before your doctor measures it. Your blood-sugar ranges might be slightly different if the normal range of your laboratory's HbA_{1C} is different from ours. Our normal range of HbA_{1C} is 4.5–6.5%. Find out your laboratory's normal HbA_{1C} range and use it to revise this table.

If you have type I diabetes, have an HbA_{1C} test done every three months.

Average Glucose	Predicted HbA_{1C}
<100	<6.5
100–120	6.5–7.0
120–140	7.0–7.5
140–160	7.5–8.0
160–180	8.0–8.5
>180	>8.5

*W*hy would my blood sugar be high
   before supper when I use regular
insulin before each meal and NPH at night?

TIP:

A verage doses of regular insulin last only 4–6 hours.
Because the time between lunch and supper can often be
6 or 7 hours, it is not surprising that your lunchtime insulin is
wearing off before supper.

An ideal insulin regimen is flexible to allow for whatever
changes come up in your day-to- day schedule. You should be
able to make adjustments to correct for unusual swings in
blood sugar that result from known or unknown causes. The
regimen you describe is very popular, but many people find
that not having an intermediate- or long-acting insulin during
the day limits how flexibile they can be. As you can see, your
regimen is not dealing with the blood sugar rise before supper.
Talk to your health-care team about this pattern you see
developing.

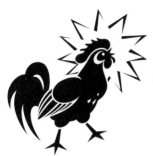

*W**hy are my morning blood sugars usually the highest of the day?*

▼
TIP:

High morning blood sugars may be caused by your insulin failing to cover your body's needs all night. In many people, NPH is too short-acting because it may last only 6–8 hours. This may not be long enough to maintain good blood-sugar levels overnight if you take your NPH at suppertime. Try moving your evening NPH injection to bedtime. If this change doesn't work, then you need to consider switching to a longer-acting insulin, such as ultralente. Many people who use two injections of ultralente per day (in addition to regular insulin before each meal) see improvement in their morning blood sugars. Or you may need to increase your dose. To see if you have nighttime lows, check your blood sugar between 2 and 4 a.m. Starting off the day with blood-sugar levels close to normal is a key to good overall blood-sugar control.

APPROXIMATE INSULIN ACTION

	Onset	Peak	Duration
Regular	<1/2 h	1–3 h	4–10 h
NPH	1–2 h	5–9 h	10–18 h
Ultralente	2–4 h	10–14 h	>24 h

Should I take large doses of regular insulin when my blood sugar is high?

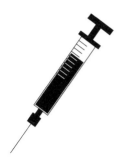

▼
TIP:

For an adult, very high blood sugars do not necessarily require very large doses of regular insulin. While increasing your insulin makes sense when your sugar is high, increasing your regular dose by more than 1 or 2 units is unlikely to make your sugar come down much faster. In fact, the main effect of taking larger dosages of regular insulin is that the insulin works over a longer period of time. A large morning dose of regular may result in mid-afternoon hypoglycemia. Thus, when your blood sugars are very high,

1 Take your regular insulin dose immediately,

2 Drink large amounts of water to stay well hydrated, and

3 Delay your next meal until your blood sugar has decreased to a level below 200 mg/dl. This may mean waiting 1 or 2 hours after injecting your insulin before eating.

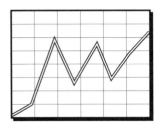

Why do my blood-sugar levels vary so much since I switched to ultralente insulin?

▼
TIP:

One of the reasons may be because you do not always get the same concentration of insulin crystals into the syringe. One basic instruction that is often overlooked when patients start on ultralente insulin is how to correctly mix the crystals. After you rock the bottle between your palms, you must immediately draw the dose out of the bottle. The weight and shape of these crystals cause them to rapidly settle back to the bottom of the bottle. If you set the bottle down to draw your regular and then return to the ultralente, the amount of insulin suspended may be quite different than if you had drawn the dose up immediately.

What should I do when it's getting close to my mealtime and my blood sugar is above 240 mg/dl?

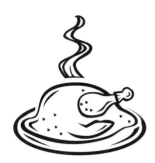

▼
TIP:

High blood sugar before a meal tells you that your liver is making too much glucose and needs to be told to slow down! The signal it needs is insulin. Because it takes time for insulin to be absorbed from the skin and more time to reduce the liver's glucose production, we suggest that you take your usual dose of insulin and wait 60–90 minutes (instead of the usual 30–45 minutes). This will allow your blood-sugar level to fall toward the normal range before you eat, giving the insulin a "head start." The goal is not to become low before eating, but to regain control over high blood sugar.

(See Tip on page 54.)

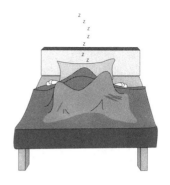

*H*ow can I sleep late on weekends without waking up with high blood sugar?

▼ TIP:

I f you want to sleep in late (for example, until 10 or 11 in the morning), then set your alarm for 6 a.m., get up, go to the bathroom, and check your blood sugar. If your blood sugar is high, take 2–4 units of regular insulin so that while you are sleeping late, your blood sugar will slowly decline. If your blood sugar is low, you should drink some juice or milk. If you are normal, take 1 or 2 units of regular insulin and go back to sleep. This schedule has worked well for many people, and often they do not even remember waking up at 6 a.m. and taking their insulin.

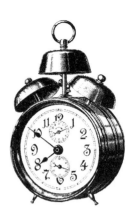

*H*ow soon after I wake up in the morning should I check my blood sugar?

▼
TIP:

C heck your blood sugar immediately upon awakening— before any morning activities, such as showering, shaving, makeup, etc. The reason for this schedule is that if your blood sugar is low, you can drink some juice or milk. If it is high, you can take your insulin immediately and allow it to work at least 1 hour before breakfast. It is important to get into this habit, because if you start the day with a normal blood-sugar level before breakfast, keeping your blood sugar under control throughout the day is much easier. Monitoring your blood sugar immediately upon awakening does not take a major change in lifestyle, but it is very effective in improving your blood-sugar control.

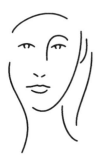

Why do my blood sugars run high before I have my menstrual period?

▼
TIP:

Many women with diabetes have swings in blood-sugar control around the time of menstruation. There are many possible reasons for this, from changes in behavior (eating more food) to hormonal changes (high estrogen levels before the period begins can increase your insulin requirements). Young women seem to have the largest swings in blood sugar during their monthly cycle, but even older women often have to adjust their insulin based on the time of the month. As you become familiar with your body's rhythm, you may find that the changes in your insulin needs are predictable from month to month. Check your blood sugar often and adjust your insulin to it during your menstrual period.

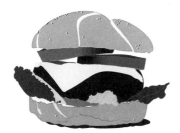

Why do I get high blood sugar after I treat a low blood-sugar reaction?

▼
TIP:

Two factors raise your blood sugar after a low blood-sugar reaction. First, the hormones (chemicals) that your body releases into your blood slowly raise the level of blood sugar. Second, the food you eat raises your blood sugar. Many people with diabetes eat or drink too much after a low blood-sugar reading. Low blood sugar causes intense hunger. All of these factors can cause high blood sugars 2–4 hours after eating. It's important to drink only a small amount (1/2 glass) of juice or milk, or eat glucose tablets, and then recheck your sugar in 30 minutes. If you eat a larger amount of food, then cover the food with extra regular insulin.

Chapter Three:
LOW BLOOD SUGAR TIPS

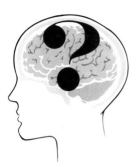

*W*ill repeated low blood sugars
damage my ability to think clearly?

▼
TIP:

W e don't know. A recent large study of people with
repeated moderate low blood sugars did not show a
decrease in the brain's functioning. But low blood-sugar levels
can be dangerous, particularly if they are very low or occur for
a prolonged period of time. The brain uses blood sugar for
energy, and if it is without fuel for longer than a few minutes,
it can suffer damage. For this reason, treat low blood sugars
rapidly, so that no damage occurs.

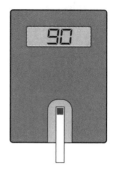

Why do I feel like my blood sugar is low when my meter says it is normal?

▼
TIP:

There are several possibilities. First, your glucose meter may be broken, dirty, or the battery may be low. Repair it, clean it, and change the battery. (Call the manufacturer if you need help.) Have your health-care team check the accuracy of your meter. Second, it takes several weeks for you to get used to normal blood sugars when you have had high blood sugars for a long period of time. Your body may be sending you false signals. Third, you can feel like your blood sugar is low if your blood sugar rapidly drops from a high level to a normal level. This usually occurs after you've taken a large dose of regular insulin. For all these reasons, don't guess what your blood sugar is—always measure it.

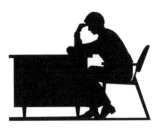

*W*hy did I have low blood sugar
this morning even though I didn't
*eat anything different and took my
usual insulin dose?*

▼
TIP:

E xercise can sometimes result in low blood sugar that night
or the next day. This is called "delayed onset low blood
sugar." A day of skiing or 18 holes of golf can result in low
blood sugar levels during your sleep that night or even the next
day. Whenever you exercise strenuously, it's a good idea to
check your blood sugar more frequently. Eat extra carbohydrates as needed during the next 24 hours, or adjust your
insulin dose.

Another factor is that intermediate- or long-acting insulin
is absorbed at different rates from day to day. You can control
this to some extent by injecting insulin into the abdominal
area, because it is absorbed better there.

A third factor may be that you forgot your nighttime snack.
This snack is important because the food you eat for supper is
usually completely absorbed by 3:00 a.m.

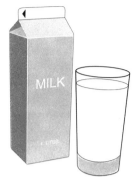

B esides glucose tablets (which I find too sweet) and juice (which I'm tired of), what other choices do I have to treat low blood-sugar reactions?

▼
TIP:

O ne of our favorite recommended treatments is a glass of milk. Milk contains lactose that is broken down to glucose (sugar). It also has fat and protein in it to slow down the rise in your blood sugar and keep it steady over time. For this reason, milk is better than juice or glucose tablets. Skim and 2% milk have the same amount of lactose. Other studies have found that a small amount of ice cream will work nearly as well. You might also consider graham crackers or a piece of bread, which are easy to keep on hand. Try to avoid high-fat treatments like candy bars, because they may lead to very high blood-sugar levels in the hours after you eat them (and can contribute to weight gain, too).

*H*ow do I protect myself against low blood sugar while I am trying for tight diabetes management?

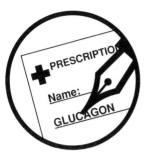

▼
TIP:

K eep glucagon handy for emergency treatment of severe low blood sugar. Glucagon raises blood sugar. In many ways it does the opposite of what insulin does. You get glucagon from the pharmacy with a prescription from your doctor. Someone in your household must know how to mix up the glucagon and inject it if you become severely hypoglycemic, confused, and unable to swallow food. This will need to be done quickly. Glucagon will raise your blood sugar within 10–15 minutes, but its effect is limited. Eat some crackers after you become fully conscious again. Some people are nauseated after receiving glucagon. Most severe reactions happen during your sleep, so to prevent your family from having to search for the glucagon, keep it in one place, such as the refrigerator door.

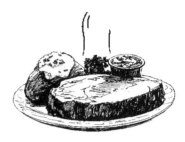

Should I take my insulin before I eat even if my blood sugar is low?

▼
TIP:

First treat the low blood-sugar level with enough food to return your blood sugar to the normal range. Liquids, rather than solids, are most rapidly absorbed and you need to drink just enough to return your blood-sugar level to normal. In 10–15 minutes, take your insulin and wait about 20 minutes before eating your meal. While this takes some willpower, it prevents your blood sugar from rebounding and ending up above your goal of a normal blood-sugar level after a meal.

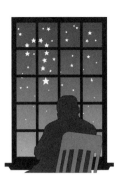

*W*hat should I do to overcome my fear
of having low blood sugar while I'm
asleep?

▼
TIP:

M any people are insecure about sleeping after having a
bad low blood-sugar reaction during the night. It is reasonable to feel fearful. Many factors influence your blood
sugar levels during the night, including how low your blood-
sugar level is before you go to sleep, exercise you did during
the day, changes in your insulin dose, and whether you ate or
skipped a nighttime snack. If you and your physician are
unable to determine why the reaction happened, try setting
your alarm to wake you at 3 a.m. several nights in a row. If
you find that you usually have a fall in your blood glucose during the night, you and your health-care provider can adjust
your evening insulin dose or bedtime snack.

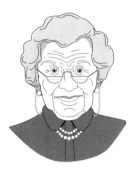

S hould my 85-year-old mother try to keep her blood sugar near 150 mg/dl instead of near the normal level of 100 mg/dl?

▼
TIP:

M aybe. She and her health-care team need to decide that. Each patient using intensified diabetes management has an individual blood glucose goal aimed at preventing the long-term complications of diabetes. However, we can say that asking people to come close to normal increases their risk of severe hypoglycemia (very low blood sugar reactions). Elderly people suffer more from low blood sugars. In fact, it may increase their risk for a heart attack or cause a stroke. For some elderly people with diabetes, the risks may outweigh the benefits of trying for normal blood-sugar levels. While 150 mg/dl is not a normal glucose concentration, it does offer your mother some room for her blood glucose to fall into the normal range with less fear of serious low blood-sugar reactions.

I live alone; what can I do to reduce the risk of a severe nighttime low blood-sugar reaction?

▼
TIP:

S tudies have shown that 50% of severe low blood-sugar reactions happen between midnight and 8 a.m. (usually at 4:00 a.m.) Having a normal blood-sugar level before you go to sleep does not guarantee that it won't drop too low a few hours later, especially if you use intensified insulin treatments, such as nighttime NPH. Test your blood-sugar level before bed and have a good bedtime snack to prevent low blood sugar before 8 a.m. If nighttime low blood sugars happen often, set your alarm and check your blood-sugar level at 3:00 a.m. every night. Eat some food if it is below 75 mg/dl.

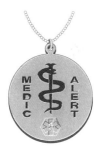

What should I do about very severe low blood-sugar episodes that cause me to pass out?

▼
TIP:

Teach your family members and friends the signs and symptoms of low blood sugar so they can help you in case you are not alert enough to tell them that your blood sugar is low. For those times when you may be someplace where no one knows you, carry a card in your wallet or wear a bracelet or necklace stating that you have diabetes. The card should also state whether you are on insulin and that you may become confused when you have low blood sugar. In this way, you may get help more quickly.

Work with your health-care team to try to determine why you are having these episodes of low blood sugar. Keep glucagon at home or with you, and be sure a family member or friend knows how to inject it for you.

Why is my blood sugar still high this evening when my low blood sugar occurred early this morning?

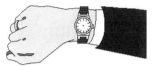

TIP:

Your body reacts to low blood sugars by secreting several hormones (chemicals), including growth hormone and cortisol. These hormones do not act immediately, but after several hours, they will raise your blood sugar. Their activity may last up to 24 hours, so you may then have to take additional insulin to keep your blood sugar from going too high. This rebound effect is one reason why you want to avoid very low blood sugars. Another reason for the high blood sugar may be that you ate too much when you tried to treat the low blood sugar reaction.

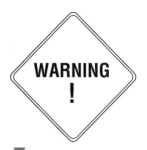

Why do I no longer feel the warning signs of low blood sugar?

▼
TIP:

Many people who have had diabetes for more than 5 years, lose some of the symptoms of low blood sugar. The usual feelings of hunger, sweatiness, anxiety, and increased heart rate may fade and escape your attention. Sometimes you may just feel sleepy as your blood sugar drops. The reasons for this are complex but are related to a loss of adrenalin release by your body when your blood sugar is low. If you are unaware of low blood sugars, try not to let your blood-sugar level drop below 100 mg/dl. You may need to monitor your blood-sugar levels more often.

If this is a problem for you, always check your blood-sugar level before you drive.

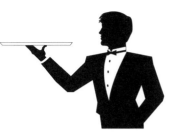

Why do I develop low blood sugar after a fancy restaurant meal?

▼

TIP:

Perhaps you prepare for a restaurant meal by injecting extra insulin. Restaurant meals are usually rich in fat and protein, but these nutrients do not raise your blood-sugar levels as quickly as carbohydrates do, and they don't require any extra insulin. In fact, a problem with restaurant meals is getting enough carbohydrates. To increase the carbohydrate content, eat well during the bread course at the start of the meal (avoiding the butter), and consider ordering a glass of skim milk with your meal or having a nonfat dessert, such as fresh fruit, or a frozen dish, such as sherbet or sorbet.

If you have an alcoholic drink when you eat out, the alcohol may be causing the low blood sugar.

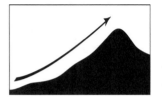

*Why do my blood sugars read
lower on my glucose meter when
I travel from Miami (sea level) to
Albuquerque (5,000 foot elevation)?*

▼
TIP:

M ost blood glucose meters use a chemical reaction that
requires oxygen from the air to measure your blood
sugar. At high altitudes there is less oxygen in the air, which
causes the results to be lower. Thus, the results you get may be
affected by altitude. You should read the instructions that came
with your meter and also read the package insert in the strips.
You may also call the 1– 800 (toll–free) number given in your
package insert or write to the company that makes your meter
to find out if its readings are affected by altitude.

Chapter Four:
INSULIN TIPS

* Please note that if you have type II diabetes
but you are taking insulin,
these tips will work for you as well.

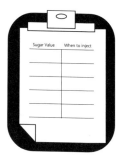

Is there a chart I can use to know how to time my insulin injections with my meals?

TIP:

Below is a schedule we provide to our patients with diabetes. The timing depends on your current blood sugar. In general, insulin should be taken 45 minutes before the meal if your blood sugar is high and at the meal if your blood sugar is low. The use of the table below should improve your after-meal blood-sugar levels.

When to Inject

If blood sugar value 45 minutes before meal is	Inject insulin:
below 50 mg/dl	when completing meal
50–70 mg/dl	at mealtime
70–120 mg/dl	15 minutes before meal
120–180 mg/dl	30 minutes before meal
over 180 mg/dl	45 minutes before meal

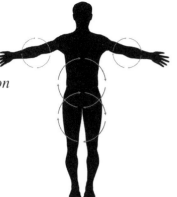

S hould I rotate my insulin injection between my arms, my legs, and abdomen?

▼
TIP:

M aybe not. True, rotating your insulin injections helps you avoid always injecting into the exact same spot on your body. You don't want to do that because insulin may cause local deposits of fat under the skin. However, insulin is absorbed at different speeds when it is injected into different areas of the body. Good blood-sugar levels depend on you knowing how quickly your insulin will act. That is why we say to rotate your injection sites in one general area—that is, arms, or legs, or around the abdomen, but not all three. You could give your morning shots in one area, and your evening shots in another area. This provides you with more predictable insulin absorption and improved blood-sugar control. We suggest using the abdomen as an injection site, because insulin is absorbed more rapidly in this location.

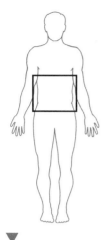

Where should I inject my regular insulin to get the most consistent absorption?

TIP:

We recommend that you use your abdomen. Insulin injected into the abdomen is absorbed quickly and predictably so you know how it will affect your blood sugar, time after time. In general there are three places to inject insulin: 1) the arms, 2) the abdomen, and 3) the legs. Several factors affect the way your body absorbs insulin. If you exercise the muscles of your arms or legs vigorously after an injection, more insulin will be absorbed more quickly. It will be difficult for you to predict how this insulin will affect your blood sugar. Warm temperatures also increase the speed at which insulin is absorbed. Because your abdomen is usually covered by clothing and stays warm, insulin is absorbed more rapidly from this area.

*H*ow long will my injection of regular
insulin last?

▼
TIP:

R egular insulin generally lasts from 3 to 6 hours. However,
the length of time that regular insulin lasts depends on the
number of units that you inject. It also depends on how sensitive you are to insulin in your blood. The more regular insulin
you inject, the longer its action lasts. One unit of insulin may
last only 1 hour, whereas 10 units of insulin may last 5 hours
or more. If you take a small dose of regular insulin before
breakfast and your blood sugar starts to rise before lunch, you
probably need to increase your dose of regular insulin before
breakfast.

What can I do about low blood sugars at 3:00 a.m. if I take my last dose of regular and NPH insulin before supper?

▼
TIP:

An easy answer is to move your NPH injection to right before bedtime. You may also need to eat a late night snack before you go to bed. Human NPH insulin has a maximum effect approximately 8–10 hours after you take it. If you take your insulin at dinnertime (6 p.m.), its peak of activity will be at about 4 a.m. Because you have also used up the food you ate at dinner by this time, you will probably have low blood sugar (hypoglycemia) at 3 a.m. When you have made adjustments to your regimen, get up at 3 a.m. and check your blood sugar level to be sure things are going as you planned.

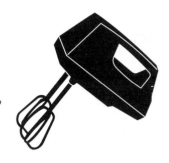

If I mix my regular insulin with my NPH or ultralente, will this reduce the effectiveness of my regular insulin?

▼
TIP:

No and yes. You can mix regular insulin with NPH insulin without altering the effect of your regular insulin. But, you cannot mix regular insulin with lente or ultralente insulin without risking some loss of regular insulin's effect. If you do choose to mix regular and ultralente, you will need to inject it immediately after mixing up the dose. It is best to take separate injections (although inconvenient) if your schedule includes regular insulin plus one of the lente insulins.

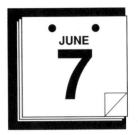

How often should I adjust the dose of my intermediate- or long-acting insulin if my blood sugar is not well-controlled?

▼
TIP:

Don't change your dose of intermediate- or long-acting insulin more often than every 3 or 4 days. Many factors affect blood-sugar levels besides insulin. Some of these factors are exercise, how much food you eat, what you eat, illness, plus the speed at which your injected insulin is absorbed. Until you have looked at these other factors, you should not adjust your intermediate- or long-acting insulin daily. Give your insulin schedule several days to work before trying a new one.

The same is true for regular insulin. You may make adjustments for a one-time high blood sugar, but changes to your regimen should come only after you've checked all the factors that affect your blood sugar level.

*H*ow *can I get my blood sugars*
under control when I have to
rotate between night and day shifts on
my job?

▼
TIP:

C learly, the best option is to negotiate with your employer to stay on one shift. The Americans with Disabilities Act requires employers to provide "reasonable accommodation for people with diabetes." Or you may want to try a more flexible insulin regimen. Using ultralente with regular insulin or an insulin pump will give you the flexibility this situation demands. One of your problems is that your body releases hormones during sleep that make insulin work less effectively. By rotating shifts, you disturb the normal release of these hormones. You don't know when the hormones are being released so you don't know how your insulin will affect your blood-sugar levels.

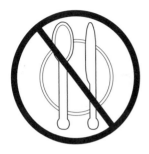

If I am using ultralente and regular insulin, do I always need to take regular insulin at lunch even if I am not going to eat?

▼
TIP:

I f your blood sugar is near normal, you probably don't need to take any additional insulin. If your blood sugar is high, you may want to take a "touchup" dose of regular at lunchtime even if you are not going to eat. Consider taking 1–5 units of regular insulin to bring your blood sugar back to normal before dinnertime. With experience, you will learn how much regular insulin to take.

What should I do if dinner is served and it has only been 15 minutes since I took my regular insulin?

▼
TIP:

Foods that are high in carbohydrates (such as bread, starches, fruit, and milk) raise blood sugar rapidly. Protein foods may be partly converted to blood sugar, but the rise in blood sugar will be much later (after the meal). Ideally, you should wait 30–45 minutes before eating for regular insulin to start working. If this is not possible, try eating first the foods that won't have much effect on blood sugar, such as the salad and meat, or sip on sugar–free drinks, such as iced tea. Save the starches, such as bread and potatoes, and eat them last so the regular insulin has another 10–15 minutes to work.

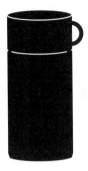

How should I store my insulin during a long car trip?

▼
TIP:

Your insulin is good at room temperature for at least 1 month. If you keep your insulin cooler than 85°F while traveling, it will be fine. If you are going to leave it in the car while you're out sightseeing, keep it in a small thermos and maybe even put the thermos in your ice chest. Don't put the bottle of insulin in direct contact with the ice in the cooler, because freezing the insulin is just as bad as overheating it. If you are camping out in winter, keep your insulin bottle in your thermos or sleeping bag.

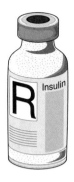

*W*hat causes my regular insulin to get
cloudy after several weeks?

▼
TIP:

A ll insulins have a tendency to change while they are
stored. Many factors speed up this change, including
warm temperatures and shaking the insulin bottle. For this
reason, you should not carry your insulin in your pocket, especially if you are an active person. Keep it in your refrigerator,
purse, cupboard, etc. to protect it from heat and motion. If
regular insulin becomes cloudy, throw it away. It has lost
effectiveness. It will not keep your blood sugar from getting
too high.

If you inject a mixture of regular and NPH insulins, you
may be getting NPH in the bottle of regular insulin. This will
make it cloudy, too.

How can I take insulin at lunch when I'm on a logging crew and can't be carrying insulin, syringes, or test supplies with me?

▼
TIP:

You could use the blood sugar monitors and injection devices that are the size and shape of pocket pens. Because you can carry these instruments in your pocket, they provide a convenient way to monitor your sugar and inject the appropriate amount of insulin at work. Your diabetes health professional can provide you with information about these devices. *Diabetes Forecast* magazine reviews the advantages and disadvantages of these devices in their October issue and in the annual *Buyer's Guide*.

If I intentionally omit my insulin dose, will I lose weight?

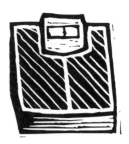

▼
TIP:

Not really. Although recent studies have suggested that some patients skip an insulin injection to lose weight, we don't recommend it. This is very hard on your system and does not accomplish your goal of fat loss. Omitting an insulin injection lets your blood sugar rise, and you lose proteins, salts, and fluid in your urine. This can make you very ill, perhaps to the point of having to be hospitalized. Do not omit your insulin injection to lose weight.

Chapter Five:
ORAL MEDICATION TIPS

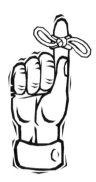

How can I remember to take my diabetes pills to prevent high blood sugars?

▼
TIP:

The best way to remember to take medication is to develop a daily routine. That is, always take the medication at the same time of day and in the same location, such as in the bathroom or at the breakfast table. To further reduce the chance of omitted medication, use a labeled pill box or pill organizer. These inexpensive boxes are available at drug stores. Set up medications in the pill box a week in advance to make it easy to know whether all your pills have been taken.The more medications you take, and the more complicated your pill-taking schedule is, the greater the likelihood that you will make mistakes. The danger of not taking diabetic medication is that your blood-sugar levels will go very high.

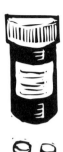

*W*hat should I do if I forget to take my diabetes pills?

▼
TIP:

If you forget to take your oral hypoglycemic agent, it is important to know whether to take it when you do remember. The rule is simple. If you are within 3 hours of the time of the dose you missed (and you normally take pills twice per day), go ahead and take your medication. If more than 3 hours have passed, wait for your next scheduled dose. Alternatively, if you are on a long-acting sulfonylurea taken once per day (glyburide or glipizide GITS) , take your medication if you are within 12 hours of missing your dose. Otherwise, wait until the next scheduled time to resume your medication.

*W*hat do you suggest that I do
when my doctor wants me to
take insulin, but I would rather take
pills for my diabetes?

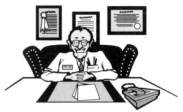

▼
TIP:

If you have type I diabetes, pills will not work for you. You
will have to take insulin injections. However, if you have
type II diabetes, then you may respond to pills. Many doctors
try pills in patients with type II diabetes, because pills are easier to take and have other advantages. Tell your doctor that you
would like to try the pills, and if they do not work, then you
would be willing to take insulin injections. There is not an
absolute "yes or no" blood test to tell how you will respond to
pills. The only way to know is to try them for several weeks
before switching to insulin injections.

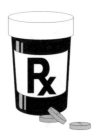

Why does my doctor want me take insulin at bedtime even though I am already taking pills for diabetes?

TIP:

Your doctor is probably concerned about your fasting (before breakfast) blood sugar being high. When pills are not keeping your fasting sugar within the normal range, it is common practice to have you take insulin at night so that your blood sugar is normal at the start of the day. You do much better with pills if your blood-sugar level before breakfast is in the normal range. If this program does not work for you, you may have to take insulin both in the morning and at night, even though you have type II diabetes.

Chapter Six:
SICK DAY TIPS

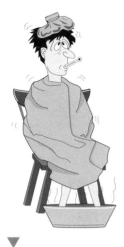

When I am ill with the flu, what should I do to keep my blood sugar from going too high?

▼
TIP:

Monitor these three factors when you are sick:

1 Your blood sugar,

2 Your urine ketones, and

3 Your body weight.

High blood sugar indicates that you need more regular insulin. High urine ketones indicate that your body needs more carbohydrates (sugar-containing drinks and more insulin) to suppress fat breakdown. A loss of weight indicates that you need more fluids. When you cannot get your blood sugar below 250 mg/dl, your urine ketones below 3+, or your body weight close to normal, then you must call your health-care team.

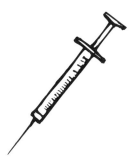

*W*hen I am sick with the flu and cannot eat food without vomiting, how do I know how much insulin to take?

▼
TIP:

The guide to how much insulin to take is your current blood sugar. You need to take enough regular insulin to keep your blood-sugar level below 200 mg/dl, so you do not become dehydrated due to excessive urination. For adults, we recommend taking an injection of at least 5 units of regular insulin every 4 hours and to keep increasing the dose of regular insulin by one unit until your blood sugar gets below 200 mg/dl. This may be more than your usual dose of insulin even though you are not eating. If you inject regular insulin every 4 hours, you should withhold your intermediate- or long- acting insulin until you get well. Of course, if you are relying solely on regular insulin, you will need to wake up during the night to take an insulin injection.

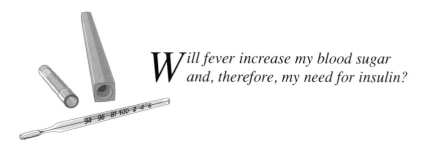

Will fever increase my blood sugar and, therefore, my need for insulin?

▼
TIP:

Yes. Even mild illness may require you to take a little more insulin. And if you develop a fever with chills, muscle aches, and sweating, you will definitely need increasing doses of insulin. In fact, your requirements of regular insulin may double. Keep a thermometer at home to determine when your body temperature is above 99°F, because this is a key to knowing when you need more insulin. You and your health-care team should develop a plan for what to do if your blood sugar is high when you are sick. Do not hesitate to call them when you are ill.

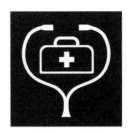

*A*t what point must I seek medical help
if I have the flu?

▼
TIP:

You should seek medical help when you cannot keep down
liquids. Contrary to popular belief, eating solid food is not
essential during short-term illness. Most people have ample
body fat stores to provide energy. However, you must be able
to drink liquids. If you are unable to hold down any fluids for
more than 12 hours, you need to seek medical help immediately. Your body will become dehydrated if you can't eat salt and
water. This can affect you seriously, causing acidosis, uncon-
sciousness, and death. Therefore, if you are vomiting all fluids
or are spilling large amounts of ketones in your urine, you
should contact your health-care team immediately.

Ideally you should set up a sick-day maintenance plan
with your health-care team before you ever get sick. That way
you will have more information about who to call and when.

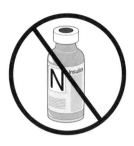

Should I skip my NPH insulin dose in the morning before a dental appointment that prevents me from eating lunch?

▼
TIP:

Not necessarily. You have two options. The first option is to omit the a.m. dose of NPH but take your regular insulin dose before you eat breakfast. You must take a dose of regular insulin about 5–6 hours after your morning dose of regular insulin (this second small dose is to keep your blood sugar under control even though you won't be eating).

The second option is to take your regular insulin and then to cut your morning NPH dose by about 1/3 (because you won't be eating lunch) and inject that. After the dental procedure (about 6 hours after your a.m. dose of regular insulin), you can take an additional small dose of regular insulin that should tide you over until dinner time.

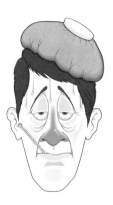

*Why are my blood sugars still high when
I had the flu a week ago?*

▼
TIP:

Major stresses cause changes in the body that may last for several weeks beyond the time when you get well. Although you may feel better now, these changes (which affect many of the substances in your body that raise blood sugar) are still active. Remember that you may need additional insulin for 1–2 weeks after a major stress (for example, severe flu, pneumonia, heart attack, etc.) in order to keep your blood-sugar levels in the normal range.

Chapter Seven:
NUTRITION TIPS

*S*hould I take vitamins or minerals to improve my blood sugar?

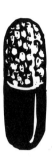

▼
TIP:

There is not enough scientific evidence to recommend vitamin or mineral supplements to improve your blood sugar. From time to time, various vitamin and mineral supplements have been popular. Recently, magnesium, chromium, zinc, vanadium, and selenium have been publicized in newspapers and promoted by health food stores.

In contrast, we strongly recommend that you get pneumonia vaccinations and annual flu vaccinations (usually available in early fall). Vaccinations may prevent (or reduce the severity of) these illnesses, which usually cause high blood sugars. Ask your health-care team for their advice.

*H*ow can I lose weight when I
hardly eat anything now?

▼
TIP:

S taying at your normal weight is one of your goals when
you are trying for normal blood sugar levels. If you are not
exercising, you will be surprised at the difference a daily
30-minute walk can make in both weight loss and blood sugar
control. Walking burns calories and lowers blood sugar. Another way to lose weight may be as simple as reducing the food
you eat by one slice of bread per day. One slice of bread contains 80 to 100 calories, and 30 slices of bread (amount eaten
in 1 month) is equal to approximately one pound of body
weight. Therefore, if you omit one of your usual slices of bread
per day for 1 year, you may lose up to 12 pounds!

If exercise becomes a daily habit, you'll need to adjust
the amount of insulin you take and the food you eat.

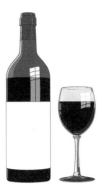

*H*ow will alcohol affect my blood sugar?

▼
TIP:

A side from the social and health problems caused by drinking too much alcohol, you have an additional concern—low blood sugar. Alcohol interferes with your body's ability to produce blood sugar and causes low blood sugar. Do not drink alcohol if you are not eating. If you are eating a meal and you drink only a small quantity of alcohol, then the alcohol should not cause you to have a severe problem with low blood sugar. You will, however, have to include the calories in the alcohol in your meal plan.

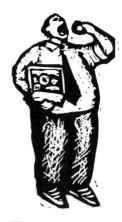

*H*ow can I lose weight and keep eating
the foods that I like?

▼
TIP:

Y ou do not have to give up all the foods that you like. It's
the size of the portion you eat that is important. Some
foods are higher in fat content than other foods. If you cut
down or cut out high-fat foods, you can lose significant
amounts of weight. To find the fat and caloric content of the
foods you eat, check paperback books listing this information
at libraries, bookstores, and pharmacies. See how much fat is
in your favorite foods. Eliminating even one high-fat food that
you eat often will result in weight loss. (Remember that exercise will help you lose weight without cutting back on any
foods.)

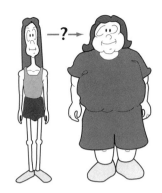

*W*ill I gain weight as I lower my blood sugar?

▼
TIP:

Not necessarily, especially if you keep track of how much you eat. However, many people do gain weight, and the reasons are complex. One factor is that you are no longer losing large quantities of calories in your urine (in the form of glucose). An equal number of calories (as was being lost in your urine) will need to be deleted from the amount of food you eat. You won't know how many calories this is unless you monitor your weight and what you eat. If you start to gain weight, reduce the amount of food you eat and exercise more. If lowering your blood sugar causes you to have more low blood sugar reactions, then the food that you eat to treat the reactions may add to a weight gain.

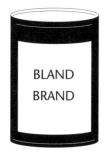

BLAND
BRAND

*W*hy don't some sugar-free foods taste very good?

TIP:

W hile some foods are actually improved by becoming "sugar-free" (canned fruit, for example), other foods are not so successfully converted to sugar-free. These are usually foods in which artificial sweeteners (sorbitol, saccharin, or aspartame) are added to taste sweet. But these sweeteners do not cook like sugar, so they don't work well in baked foods and may leave a bitter aftertaste. Also remember that these foods are not necessarily low in calories. For example, sugar-free pudding made with 2% milk has 90 calories per serving compared with 140 calories per serving for regular pudding. Although 90 is less than 140, it still isn't "calorie-free." You don't have to eat only sugar-free cookies. You may have a "real" cookie as long as it is included in your meal plan.

*H*ow large a snack should I eat at bedtime?

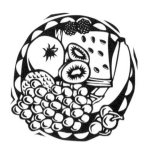

▼
TIP:

You should eat about 1/7 of your total calories per day before you go to sleep if you have a normal blood-sugar level. Your bedtime snack is designed to keep enough glucose in your blood so that your blood sugar does not get too low in the middle of the night. The NPH or ultralente insulin you took before supper can "peak" during this time and cause low blood sugar. Your health-care team can help you adjust your snack to work with your insulin or medication dose so that your morning blood sugar will be in the normal range. A snack may not be necessary if your bedtime blood sugar is over 180 mg/dl. If your bedtime blood sugar is less than 180 mg/dl, you will probably want to have a snack that includes starch and protein, such as peanut butter and crackers or low-fat cheese on toast. You may need to add a glass of skim milk or a serving of fruit if your blood sugar is less than 100 mg/dl.

BEDTIME SNACK SUMMARY

Blood Sugar	Snack Quantity
<100 mg/dl	juice and usual snack
101–180 mg/dl	usual snack
>181 mg/dl	no snack

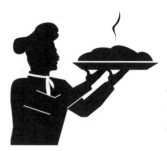

My goal is to be normal weight with near normal blood sugars, so how do I reduce fat in a meal when I eat at a restaurant?

▼ TIP:

Meat is the best place to start cutting fat calories. If you order fish that is broiled or baked, it will usually have less than 5 grams of fat per ounce. If you order a meat serving from the menu, look for foods that are grilled or broiled. Also look for a lower fat meat such as sirloin, instead of prime rib or filet. Ask the waiter how many ounces there are in the serving size. You may even be able to request a particular serving size, such as "bring only a 4-ounce serving of the sirloin," or request that the meat be prepared with no fat. Other sources of fat are gravies and sauces. If in doubt, request the sauce on the side and check it out before you find your chicken breast swimming in butter. Meats that are processed, such as bratwurst, lunch meats, and sausages, can be very high in fat (as much as 10–15 grams per ounce) and are usually very high in salt as well.

*H*ow can I have orange juice for
breakfast without risking high
blood sugars later?

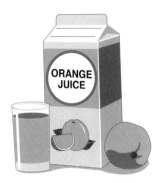

▼
TIP:

It is better for you to eat the orange (or any other fruit) than
to drink the juice from that fruit. If you like the bright wake-
up taste of orange juice first thing in the morning, try a sugar-
free citrus flavored drink mix. You will get the orange tangy
taste without any sugar! It isn't so much the sugar in the
orange but the liquid form that makes orange juice (or any
other juice) raise your blood sugar rapidly. Studies comparing
juice and sugar-containing soft drinks found there is no difference in the effect they have on people's blood sugar. We advise
people to use juice as "treatment" for low blood sugar, not as
food.

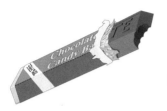

Can I eat candy bars now that the ADA is including table sugar in the diabetic diet?

▼
TIP:

Sometimes. It is true that the most recent dietary guidelines for people with diabetes include simple sugars, including table sugar. Several studies have shown that table sugar eaten as part of a meal plan does not have any worse effect on blood glucose than rice or potatoes. This does not mean, however, that people with diabetes can eat sweets freely. Sugars must be included as part of your meal plan. And the reason you still want to limit the number of candy bars you eat is that most of the calories in candy bars come from fat. Fat should be limited in everybody's diet!

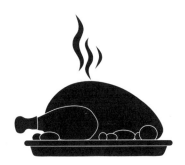

How can I keep my blood sugar normal during the holidays when high-calorie, high-fat foods are served?

▼
TIP:

Holidays are always difficult because of the change in daily routine and the increased availability of high-calorie, high-fat foods. We recommend three approaches to preventing your hemoglobin A_{1C} from rising during the holidays. First, a week before the holiday, try to control your blood sugars so that any indulgences during the holiday will be balanced by these better than usual blood-sugar levels. Second, make it a point never to eat between scheduled meals, even if cakes and cookies are available. Sticking to standard mealtimes will keep your insulin injections on schedule and prevent high blood sugars. Third, never accept second portions at any meal, even though they are offered. Simply tell your host that you are full. Don't let the holidays disturb your blood-sugar control, and you'll feel better during and after the festivities. Fourth, exercise more. Take a walk! Fifth, if you do eat more than usual, adjust your insulin.

Chapter Eight:
EXERCISE TIPS

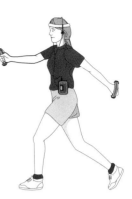

*H*ow can I get the regular exercise that
I need to improve my blood sugar?

▼
TIP:

W alk. Many people are surprised to learn that walking is
an excellent exercise. We recommend walking for
everyone. You burn approximately 200 calories in a 1 hour
walk. You will lose one pound every 2 1/2 weeks from this 1
hour of exercise (providing that you don't increase the amount
of food you eat). Walk to the shopping center, the supermarket,
or the corner drugstore instead of driving. Walking is easy on
the muscles and joints and rarely causes low blood sugar.
Exercise may make your body more sensitive to insulin so it
can help you achieve a normal body weight and a normal
blood-sugar level. Start walking today!

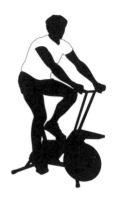

*D*oes exercise raise or lower my blood sugar?

▼
TIP:

E xercise will either raise or lower your blood sugar depending on how much insulin is in your blood. Muscles use glucose, so your blood-sugar level gets lower during exercise. This level will go even lower if there is a lot of insulin in your blood. But, you must have some insulin circulating in your blood or, in response to exercise, your liver will make more glucose, causing your blood-sugar level to rise.

Check your blood sugar before you exercise. If it is low, you can drink a sugar-containing beverage. If it is high, you can take a small dose of regular insulin. The more intense the exercise, the more difficult it is to predict whether your blood sugar will increase or decrease. If you exercise for a long time, recheck your blood sugar halfway through. With experience, you will be able to predict how your exercise will affect your blood-sugar levels.

How much food do I need to eat to avoid low blood sugars when I exercise?

▼
TIP:

The amount of food needed to prevent low blood sugar during or after exercise is different for each person. In general, if your blood sugar is below 150 mg/dl before exercising, having a snack of 15 grams of carbohydrate is a good idea (one fruit serving, one starch serving). If you have problems with low blood sugars much later after exercise, have a snack of 15–30 grams of carbohydrate within 30 minutes of finishing the exercise to help your body replace the glucose normally stored in muscle and to prevent low blood sugar later. This could be a sandwich, 5–10 saltine crackers, or 4–8 vanilla wafers or animal crackers. If you are exercising immediately before or after a meal, you may be able to reduce the regular insulin used for meal coverage, because the exercise will reduce the blood sugar that normally increases following a meal.

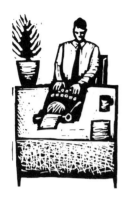

Why do I get low blood sugar when I mow the lawn on Saturday morning but never when I'm at my desk during the week?

▼
TIP:

Muscles use blood glucose to do work, so if you eat the same amount of food and take the same dose of insulin, you can expect your blood sugar will be lower on the day when you are more physically active. You have four choices:

1 Eat more carbohydrate with breakfast,

2 Decrease your morning dose of regular insulin (about 20–40% less is usually needed to allow for an hour of yard work),

3 Eat a mid-morning snack to prevent the hypoglycemia (low blood sugar level), or

4 Let your grass grow.

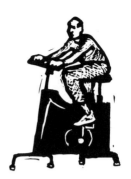

*W*hy does my blood sugar get low in the middle of the night after I exercise during the day?

▼
TIP:

E xercise is good for you, but it can bring on low blood sugar in several ways. Exercise helps you use insulin more efficiently so that a given amount of insulin has more blood-sugar–lowering power. These effects of exercise can last for up to 24 hours after the exercise has ended. That's why insulin doses should usually be decreased before and after exercise. Also, you should eat a meal or have a snack before exercising if your blood sugar is normal or low. If you balance your insulin, your food intake, and your exercise, you will have fewer low blood sugars during the night after your daytime exercise.

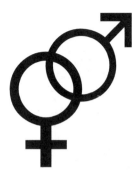

Why do I sometimes seem to get low blood sugar after having sex?

▼
TIP:

Sex is just as much an exercise as jogging or aerobics. Planning to eat food either immediately before or shortly after exercise to cover the glucose that you use is the way to avoid low blood sugar. You may want to check your blood sugar first, even though it may reduce the spontaneity of the moment. You might also consider increasing your snack before going to bed.

Chapter Nine:
EDUCATIONAL TIPS

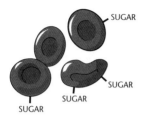

SUGAR

SUGAR

SUGAR

SUGAR

W̶hat is the "glycosylated hemoglobin test"?

▼
TIP:

The glycosylated hemoglobin test measures the percentage of hemoglobin molecules (the chemical in our blood that carries oxygen) that have sugar attached to them. Because this percentage directly reflects the average blood-sugar levels over the life of a red blood cell (90 days), this information helps you and your health-care team assess your overall blood-sugar control. There are several different tests that are used to measure glycosylated hemoglobin (such as a test called "hemoglobin A_{1C}"), and each test has its own normal range and target values. Ask your doctor what test he or she is using and what the target value should be for you. The glycosylated hemoglobin test, along with self blood-sugar monitoring, has made good blood-sugar control possible for people with diabetes.

Where can I find new information that will help me with my blood-sugar management?

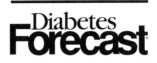

▼
TIP:

There are several ways to find out about new discoveries and products that will help you control your blood-sugar levels. First, check to see if your state American Diabetes Association (ADA) affiliate has a chapter near you. They have meetings and discussions about new products and techniques to treat diabetes. Second, you can subscribe to *Diabetes Forecast* magazine published by ADA. This magazine has many tips that will help you keep up to date. ADA has other publications about diabetes (see Resources). Third, there are now many professionals who specialize in diabetes care (certified diabetes educators—CDE) with a wealth of information about diabetes. Ask your doctor to recommend a diabetes educator/nurse to help you manage your diabetes. Or you can call the American Association of Diabetes Educators at (800)TEAM-UP4 for a list of Certified Diabetes Educators in your area.

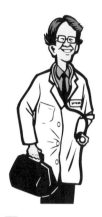

*S*hould I see a diabetes specialist for my
diabetes care?

▼
TIP:

I n the U.S., 80% of people with diabetes see physicians who
are family practice or general practice physicians. If you
feel you are getting your blood-sugar levels into the goal range
and have a good relationship with your doctor, you do not need
a diabetes specialist. Sometimes your family doctor will refer
you to a specialist for occasional visits or a "consultation" to
get some help with managing your diabetes, but then you can
continue your routine care with your family physician. If your
primary-care doctor can't help you with the daily activities of
living with diabetes, you may benefit from diabetes education.
(See Resources for the American Association of Diabetes Educators.)

How often should I see my doctor to keep my blood sugar under control?

CALENDAR			
JANUARY	FEBRUARY ✔	MARCH	APRIL
MAY ✔	JUNE	JULY	AUGUST ✔
SEPTEMBER	OCTOBER	NOVEMBER ✔	DECEMBER

▼
TIP:

As you tighten control of your diabetes, you will need to see your doctor weekly or every two weeks, at first. How often you see your doctor or diabetes educator will depend on how long you have had diabetes, your ability to adjust your insulin regimen for tight blood-sugar control, and whether you have any diabetic complications or other medical problems that may interfere with your diabetes management. After that, a visit every three months may be enough to reach your target goals.

At a minimum, you should plan on seeing your doctor twice a year to arrange for necessary eye and kidney check-ups and to stay motivated about good blood-sugar control. You should have someone you can contact on short notice to discuss problems as they arise, such as unexplained high blood sugars or sudden illness. This person does not have to be a physician but may be a certified diabetes educator, nurse practitioner, or nurse case manager.

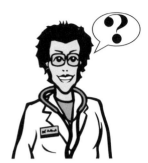

*W*hy does my doctor ask me about the
average blood sugar reading on my
monitor?

▼
TIP:

Y**ou** can use the average blood sugar that your meter calcu-
lates to improve your blood-sugar control. These averages
are not a true average of your blood-sugar levels, but only an
average of the times you've actually tested. (If, like most people with diabetes, you measure your blood sugar before meals
and at bedtime, this value could more accurately be called your
"average premeal blood sugar.") People with diabetes with
good blood-sugar control maintain this average blood sugar
below 140 mg/dl. If your average is much higher than this,
then you know that you need to adjust your diabetes management program.

*H*ow does the glycosylated
hemoglobin or hemoglobin
A_{1C} (*HbA*$_{1C}$) help me monitor my
blood-sugar control?

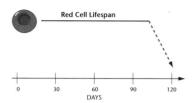

▼
TIP:

G lycosylated hemoglobin and hemoglobin A_{1C} are names
for tests that measure how much glucose (blood sugar) is
attached to your red blood cells. This interaction with glucose
occurs slowly and becomes permanent over time. Because a
red blood cell stays in your body approximately 120 days,
measuring how much glucose is attached to your red blood
cells is a good indication of your average blood sugar over a 2-
to 4- month period. It cannot, however, tell whether you are
having frequent ups and downs in your blood-sugar levels.
Studies have shown that the lower your glycosylated hemoglobin or hemoglobin A_{1C}, the less likely you are to have many of
the problems caused by diabetes.

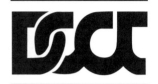

What is the "DCCT" and how does it affect me?

▼
TIP:

The DCCT is the Diabetes Control and Complications Trial, a long-term diabetes study that proved that the complications of diabetes can be delayed or prevented by good blood-sugar control. More than 1,400 people with type I diabetes were enrolled in this study at centers all across America for a period of 5–8 years. Half of these people received "conventional" diabetes care (one to two insulin injections per day) and half received "intensive" diabetes management (as many injections as necessary to maintain near-normal blood sugar). People in the intensive therapy group had significantly fewer diabetes complications. As a result of the DCCT, everyone with diabetes (type I or II) should be working to keep their blood-sugar levels closer to normal.

Decreased risk in the Intensive Therapy Group of the DCCT

Diabetic eye disease	76% decreased risk
Diabetic kidney disease	54% decreased risk
Diabetic nerve disease	60% decreased risk

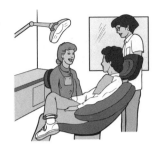

H ow does the health of my teeth
   affect my blood-sugar control?

▼
TIP:

C hronic gum disease can be a cause of unexplained high
  blood sugars. People with diabetes should have their teeth
professionally cleaned at least twice a year, because they have a
much higher risk of developing gum disease than people without diabetes. Gum disease results from the formation of plaque
underneath the gum line after eating. Plaque hardens into tartar,
which irritates the gums and gradually erodes the underlying
bone that holds the teeth in place. Thus, gum disease can lead to
the need for dentures. Daily dental care can prevent gum disease from getting started. Brush your teeth at least twice a day
with a soft-bristled brush and floss daily. Flossing removes food
from between the teeth and plaque from the gum line.

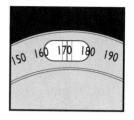

*W*hy have I gained 15 pounds over the 3 years that I have been working to improve my blood-sugar control?

▼
TIP:

S ome people who practice "intensified management" to keep their diabetes under control gain weight. Because insulin is a hormone that helps your body process the food you eat, one of its actions is to store fat. It makes sense, then, that injecting insulin to keep your blood sugar down will also result in increased fat storage. The reasons you want good blood-sugar control (for example, a decreased risk of eye and kidney disease) are usually more important than this potential weight gain. The best way to avoid gaining weight is to develop an active lifestyle and follow your health-care team's recommended meal plan, limiting fat and total calories.

*H*ow can I encourage my child to take insulin injections if he or she is scared to death of needles?

▼
TIP:

Try one of the insulin injection devices that do not use needles. They inject insulin by squirting it into the skin at high pressure. Many people with "needlephobia" prefer this method of insulin delivery. Blood-sugar control with these devices is as good or better than that achieved with syringe-injected insulin. Although cumbersome and expensive, one of these devices used for a few weeks or months may help your child to become more comfortable with the process so that he or she will be willing to try using the syringe to inject the insulin.

You could also try one of the insertion aids that hide the needle from view and help you give the injection more quickly. If the child continues to be afraid, he or she may need to talk to a mental health specialist.

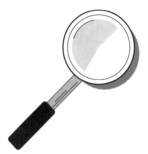

My eyesight is very poor— how can I read the numbers on my glucose meter and then correctly fill my syringe?

▼
TIP:

Many people with diabetes have visual problems. For this reason, there are blood glucose meters that also announce your results. You will be able to check the numbers you can see against the numbers you can hear. To read the numbers on your insulin syringe, you can use a magnifying glass, or buy a magnifier that fits on the syringe. You might also consider using a pen-like insulin injector that gives a specific amount of insulin with each click, which you hear as you push the plunger. Your doctor or the American Diabetes Association can provide you with information on both of these devices. (See Resources.)

Chapter Ten:
RESOURCES

Manufacturers listed in this section
can provide tips for proper use of their products.

To request more information about other books published by the American Diabetes
Association, write to:
American Diabetes Association
1970 Chain Bridge Road
McLean, VA 22109-0592

American Association of Diabetes Educators . . . . . .(800) 338-3633
444 N. Michigan Ave. . . . .(312) 644-2233
Suite 1240
Chicago, IL 60611-3901

American Diabetes Association . . . .(800) 232-3472
1660 Duke Street . . . .(703) 549-1500
Alexandria, VA 22314

American Dietetic Association . . . .(800) 366-1655
216 West Jackson Blvd.
Suite 800
Chicago, IL 60606-6995

Becton Dickinson Consumer Products . . . .(800) 237-4554
One Becton Drive
Building #2
Franklin Lakes, NJ 07417-1883

Boehringer Mannheim Corporation . . . .(800) 858-8072
9115 Hague Rd.
P.O. Box 50100
Indianapolis, IN 46250-0100

Chronimed, Inc. . . . .(800) 444-5951
Ridgedale Office Center, Suite 250 . . . .(612) 541-0239
13911 Ridgedale Dr.
Minneapolis, MN 55305

Disetronic Medical Systems, Inc.
13005 16th Avenue North, Suite 500 . . . .(800) 688-4578
Plymouth, MN 55441 . . . .(612) 551-1941

Eli Lilly and Company . . . .(800) 545-5979
Lilly Corporate Center . . . .(317) 276-2000
Indianapolis, IN 46285

Home Diagnostics, Inc . . . .(800) 342-7226
51 James Way . . . .(908) 542-7788
Eatontown, NJ 07724

International Diabetes Center . . . .(612) 927-3393
13911 Redgedale Dr.
Minnetonka, MN 55447

International Diabetic Athletes Association . . . .(602) 230-8155
6829 North 12th Street, Suite 205
Phoenix, AZ 85014

101 Tips For Improving Your Blood Sugar

Joslin Diabetes Center . . . .(617) 732-2415
Communications Office
One Joslin Place
Boston, MA 02215

Juvenile Diabetes Foundation . . . .(800) 223-1138
432 Clark Ave., South
16th Floor
New York, NY 10016

Lifescan, Inc. . . . .(800) 227-8862
1000 Gilbraltar Drive . . . .(408) 263-9789
Milpitas, CA 95035-6312

Medic Alert Foundation . . . .(800) 432-5378
PO Box 1009
Turlock, CA 95381-1009

MediSense, Inc. . . . .(800) 527-3339
266 Second Ave.
Waltham, MA 02154

Miles, Inc. (Ames) . . . .(800) 348-8100
P.O. Box 70
Elkhart, IN 46515

Minimed Technologies . . . .(800) 933-3322
12744 San Fernando Rd.
Sylmar, CA 91342

National Chronic Pain Outreach Association . . . . .(301) 652-4948
7979 Old Georgetown Road, Suite 100 . . . .(301) 907-0745 (fax)
Bethesda, MD 20814

National Diabetes Information Clearinghouse . . . . .(301) 468-2162
Box NDIC
9000 Rockville Pike
Bethesda, MD 20892

Novo Nordisk Pharmaceuticals, Inc . . . .(800) 727-6500
100 Overlook Center . . . .(609) 987-5800
Suite 200
Princeton, NJ 08540

The Upjohn Company . . . .(800) 253-8600
7000 Portage Road . . . .(616) 323-4000
Kalamazoo, MI 49001

INDEX

A
Abdomen, insulin injections in, 55–56
Absorption, of insulin, 55–56
ACE inhibitors, 13
Adrenalin, 50
Age factors, 19, 46
Alcohol (beverage), 83
Alcohol (rubbing), sterilizing skin, 11
Altitude, glucose meter readings and, 52
American Association of Diabetes Educators, 101–102
American Diabetes Association, 5, 101
Americans with Disabilities Act, 61
Amputations, 26
Arms, insulin injections in, 55
Arterial hardening, 9
Artificial sweeteners, 86
Aspartame, 86
Average blood sugar levels, 3, 6, 17, 27, 104

B
Bedtime snacks, 41, 87, 98
Blindness, 26
Blood pressure
  excess weight and, 18
  medication for, 13
  records of, 6
Blood sugar levels
  age and, 19, 46
  average, 3, 6, 17, 27, 104
  blood pressure and, 13, 18
  complications and, 9, 17, 19, 103, 106
  for elderly persons, 19, 46
  excess weight and, 18
  exercise and. *See* Exercise
  eye disease and, 10
  fasting, 72
  glycosylated hemoglobin and. *See* Glycosylated hemoglobin
  goals for, 4–5
  hemoglobin and. *See* Hemoglobin
  high. *See* Hyperglycemia
  improving, 8–9
  insulin pumps and, 15, 61

H
Halos, seeing, 25
Health-care teams, 24, 40, 74, 77, 81, 87
Heart problems, 9, 26, 46
Hemoglobin, 4–5
  A$_{1C}$, 4–5, 17, 28, 91, 100, 105
  glycosylated, 5, 100, 105
Holidays, nutrition and, 91
Hormones, 37, 43, 49, 61
Human insulin, 30, 32, 58
Hunger, 25
Hyperglycemia, 22–37, 89
  complications of, 26
  and dinner, 29
  following hypoglycemia, 49
  and foot pain, 23
  glycosylated hemoglobin and, 27
  gum disease and, 107
  health care teams and, 24
  hypoglycemic reactions and, 37
  and large insulin doses, 31
  meals and, 33
  menstrual periods and, 36
  morning, 30
  sickness and, 74, 79
  sleeping late and, 34
  symptoms of, 25
Hypoglycemia, 4, 8, 12, 17, 37–52
  alcohol and, 83
  brain damage and, 39
  elderly persons and, 46
  exercise and, 41, 95, 97
  fainting and, 48
  hyperglycemia following, 49
  insulin with, 44
  intensified diabetes management and, 43, 46
  morning, 41
  nighttime, 45, 47, 58, 97
  perceived vs. actual, 40
  physical activity and, 96
  pre-meal, 44
  reactions. *See* Reactions, hypoglycemic
  restaurant meals and, 51
  sexual activity and, 98
  thinking ability and, 39

warning signs, 50

I
Identification cards, diabetes patient, 48
Illness. *See* Sickness
Infections, 26
Information, sources of, 101
Injection points, 41, 55–56
Injections, children and, 109
Injection timing, 54
Injectors, pen-like, 66, 110
Insulin, 33
 absorption of, 55–56
 cloudiness of, 65
 doses. *See* Doses, insulin
 effectiveness of, 59, 93, 97
 human, 30, 32, 58
 with hypoglycemia, 44
 injection points, 41, 55–56
 injection timing, 54
 intentional omission of, 67
 intermediate-acting. *See* Intermediate-acting insulin
 lente, 59
 long-acting. *See* Long-acting insulin
 NPH. *See* NPH insulin
 occupational constraints on use, 66
 oral medication. *See* Oral medication
 regimens, 61
 regular. *See* Regular insulin
 resistance to, 18
 storage of, 64
 tips, 53-67
 ultralente, 30, 32, 59, 61–62, 87
Insulin-Dependent Diabetes Mellitus (IDDM), 2, 4, 20, 71, 106
Insulin injectors, pen-like, 66, 110
Insulin pumps, 15, 61
Insurance, 15
Intensified diabetes management, 19, 43, 46, 103, 106, 108
Intermediate-acting insulin, 16, 29, 41, 60, 75

J
Job shift changes, 61
Juice, 34, 42

K
Kidney disease, 9, 13, 18, 26, 106

L
Lactose, 42
Legs
  insulin injections in, 55
  pain in, 23
Lente insulin, 59
Liquids, 89
Long-acting insulin, 16, 29, 41, 60, 75, 79
Lunch. *See* Meal(s)

M
Meal(s), 3–5, 27, 44, 60. *See also* Nutrition; Snacks
  alcoholic beverages with, 83
  breakfast, 3, 27, 57, 89, 96
  delaying, 31
  dinner, 27, 29, 63
  glycosylated hemoglobin and, 27
  hyperglycemia and, 33
  insulin injection timing and, 54
  insulin pumps and, 15
  lunch, 27, 57, 62, 66, 78
  plans, 24
  pre-exercise, 97
  restaurant, 51, 88
  schedule of, 16, 91
Medical help, 77. *See also* Health-care teams; Physicians
Medications, 24
Menstrual periods, hyperglycemia and, 36
Meters, blood glucose, 14, 40, 52, 104
Microalbuminuria, 13
Milk, 34, 42, 51, 87
Money, saving, 7
Morning hyperglycemia, 30
Morning hypoglycemia, 41
Mornings, checking blood-sugar levels in, 35

N
Needlephobia, 109
Nerve disease, 9, 21, 26, 106
Nighttime hypoglycemia, 45, 47, 58, 97
Nighttime insulin, with oral medication, 72
Non-Insulin–Dependent Diabetes Mellitus (NIDDM), 2, 5, 20,

71–72, 106
NPH insulin, 29–30, 47, 58–59, 78, 87
Nurse case managers, 103
Nurse practitioners, 103
Nutrition, 80–91. *See also* Meal(s)
  alcoholic beverages and, 83
  bedtime snacks, 41, 87
  candy bars, 90
  holiday, 91
  restaurant meals, 51, 88
  sugar-free foods, 86
  vitamins and minerals, 81
  weight gain and, 85
  weight loss and, 82, 84

O
Occupational constraints, insulin use and, 66
Oral medication, 68–72
  daily routines for, 69
  forgetting, 70
  insulin vs., 71
  insulin with, 72
Orange juice, 89

P
Pen-like insulin injectors, 66, 110
Pen-like insulin monitors, 66
Physical activity, 24, 96, 108. *See also* Exercise
Physicians, 9, 28, 43, 71–72, 77, 100, 102–104
Pills. *See* Oral medication
Pneumonia vaccinations, 81
Protein foods, 63

R
Reactions, hypoglycemic, 37, 42–43, 46–47
Rebound effect, 49
Records, diabetes management and, 6
Regular insulin, 16, 30–31, 34, 40, 56–59, 61–63, 65, 75–76, 78, 94–96
Restaurant meals, 51, 88

S
Saccharin, 86
Sexual activity, 26, 98
Sickness, 60, 73–79

Urination, frequent, 25
Urine ketones, 4, 74, 77

V
Vaccinations, 81
Vision problems, 25–26, 110
  eye disease, 9–10, 106
Vitamins and minerals, 81
Vomiting, 75, 77

W
Waking, checking blood-sugar levels upon, 35
Walking, 82, 93
Warning signs, of hypoglycemia, 50
Weight
  excess, 18
  gain, 8, 42, 85, 108
  loss, 67, 82, 84, 93
  maintenance, 88
  monitoring, 6
Well-being, feelings of, 9
  records of, 6